Read this BEFORE your Knee Replacement Surgery!

By

Barbara L. Boyer

This is an informational book for the purpose of educating anyone who is considering
a knee replacement.

It is not a medical guide, but a recount of facts that happened to me.

I write this with the hope that it can be used to help anyone who is on the fence about an impending knee replacement, has or is having a similar experience and want to know they are not alone.

There are 10,000 baby boomers retiring everyday.

A lot of these people have a need to get their knees replaced and have been in pain for a million different reasons.

There are a myriad of things you should know about and consider taking care of, in preparation for your surgery.

It's a very scary thought when you learn what can happen to you… and, I know this situation first hand. You owe it to yourself and your people to read about it and then make an informed decision before going ahead with your surgery.

1) I suggest you ask your Doctor about your risk of a **staph infection** and if you should be given antibiotics before and after your surgery.

2)   1-2 % of patients become infected with staph infections after knee surgery.

3)   The most common one is staphylococcus aureus, which is a bacteria that lives on your skin and cannot be seen by the naked eye. There is nothing you can do to get rid of it… ever.

4)   Infectious Disease Doctors are now (as of 2016) anticipating the rise of staph infections to hit 15 people out of a hundred, who receive knee replacements, by 2021. This does not count hips, shoulders, etc.

5)   There are numerous ways this bacteria can enter your body, but it usually occurs at the time of surgery, although, mine happened ten months after my knee replacement. (I know a man who contracted his staph infection 10 years after his knee replacement. Another woman who was in

physical therapy with me, contracted it 5yearsafter hers.)

In my case, my immune system dropped and I contracted a case of shingles, even though I had received a shingles shot. Luckily I was not in severe pain, but I had small blisters and felt like something was crawling under my skin. But other than that, I did not feel sick... just a little off for a few weeks prior to what happened to me next.

We think, but do not know for sure, that the bacteria entered into my body and then into my blood stream, through the blisters from the shingles.

It apparently headed straight for my new knee... because there is no blood flow in the joint and the metal and plastic are essentially unprotected. Bacteria love those kinds of places inside the human body...they are all warm and it's dark and they breed by the billions in that kind of an environment.

So, ten months after I my first knee replacement, I found myself not being able to stand up from a sitting position, or bend my leg. My knee joint was swollen to the size of a cantaloupe, bright pink and very hot to the touch.

I could not get into our truck so the Paramedics took me to the hospital. From there, I was tested for an infection and put on broad-spectrum antibiotics until they could grow the bacteria in the lab to verify what type of infection I had.

In the mean time, I was given two pints of blood.

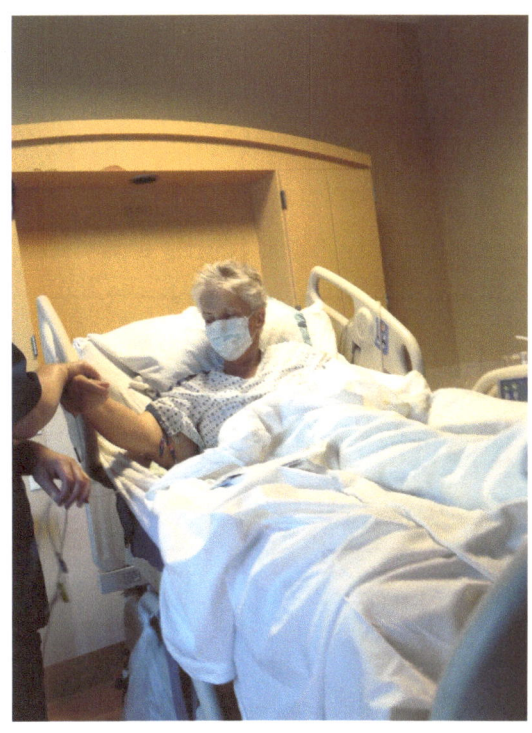

I was on blood thinner and they had to take me off
of it and fill me full of vitamin K to thicken my
blood, so I would not bleed to death on the
surgery table.

Then, when my blood test results proved right,
my Surgeon removed my knee joint, cleaned out
the entire area and placed an antibiotic spacer
where my knee joint had been. The surgery took 5
½ hours.

… I had been so happy with my original new knee. We walked every day, went to Disneyland, were able to ride on our son's boat, etc. It was a gift from the heavens and I was able to do most of the things I had not been able to do for years…

But there I was, caught in this unexpected, never thinking anything "like this could happen to me" situation, with huge unknowns facing my husband and myself.

After the surgery, I spent several days in the hospital and was then transferred to a long-term care facility, where I spent seven weeks receiving three bags of antibiotics per day, via a pic line. My Surgeon indicated that if it had been any worse I could have spent a year in ICU.

I had my useless leg in a full-length unbendable brace, until the infection was determined to be gone. The antibiotics made me nauseous and I threw up all the time. My hair was falling out by small handfuls. I lost thirty-five pounds.

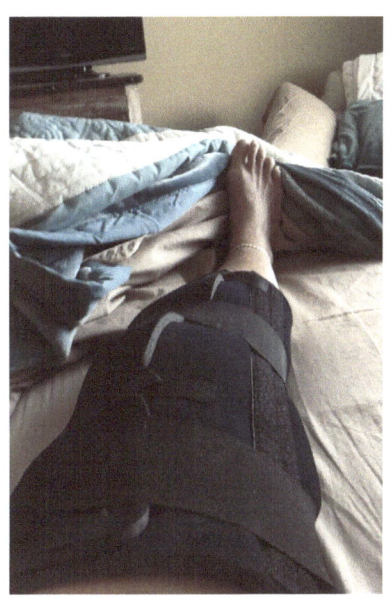

I was then transferred to my home by ambulance, and each day I had to travel by special taxi that allowed me to sit in my wheel chair with my leg extended out in front of me to the Infusion Center. For 10 more days, I received one bag of antibiotic per day. Each bag of antibiotics was $4,700.

All during this time my husband was by my side, providing all of my meals, giving me bed baths, passing out additional meds, moral support and changed the sheets on my rented hospital bed every day. He kissed me on my forehead, held my hand, told me how well I was doing, etc. My family traveled to see me, and coached me on staying positive.

The antibiotics caused me to get C-diff and my knee revision surgery had to be postponed until we could get that cleared up.

So, three months after my original knee joint removal, I went back into the hospital for my knee revision, at which time, I received a Stryker Triathlon appliance that has a hinge in the back and rods that extend down into my tibia and up into my femur.

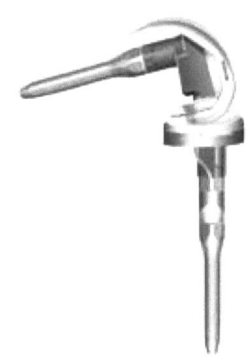

My Infectious Disease Doctor has placed me on Doxycycline 100mg twice a day <u>for life</u>. The type of antibiotic and dosages may have to be adjusted as we go along, because I run a 50/50 chance of contracting another staph infection and the Doxy may become ineffective.

My Surgeon stated that if I do get another staph infection, he will have to amputate my leg because he had to cut away so much of my bacteria eaten leg bones. You can see how much muscle had to be taken.

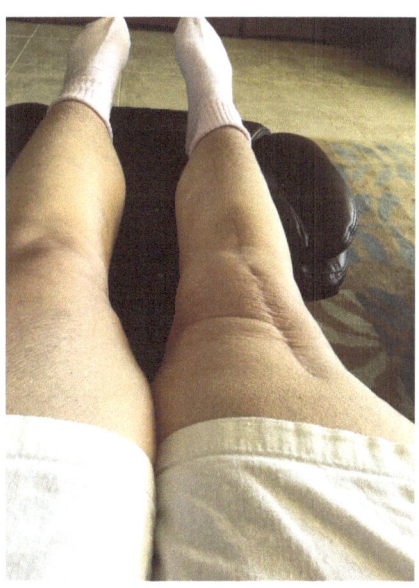

Because I am a Senior Citizen, I am on Medicare and as near as we can tell, Medicare has paid out $1.4 million, just on this one leg. There are items I needed for which they refused to pay. So our out of pocket was somewhere around $3,000 to $5,000.

My Infectious Disease Doctor explained my situation thusly:

"It was just your turn."

Really? I was dumbfounded. Until that spoint I kept trying to figure out what I had done wrong. I justified my behavior as a person who showers at least once a day, wears clean clothes, constantly washes my hands, etc., etc. But the staph bacteria, has one purpose and one purpose only… to find a way to live. Apparently without a way to naturally fight it off, my knee replacement had been a perfect host.

As my revision progressed, I was allowed to graduate to a brace that allowed me to re-learn how to bend my knee in increments of degrees: 30, then 60, then 90, then 110.

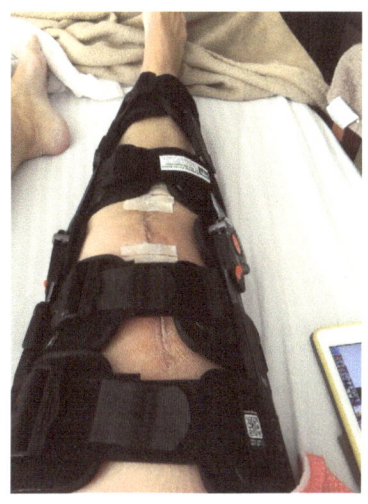

I have gone through an emotional roller coaster, (at one point my husband asked me if I wanted a turkey sandwich and I sobbed for a half hour.) I believe I had/have a minor case of PTSD. This kind of thing can't happen to me… but, it can and it did. And it could happen to anybody.

I was pretty sick. **But here I am now**

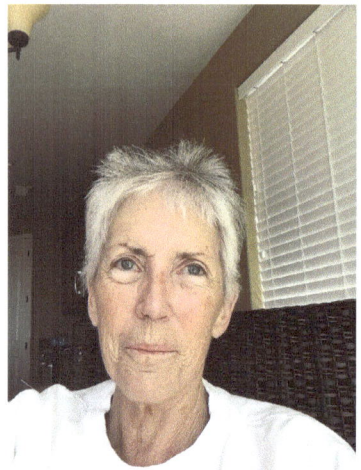 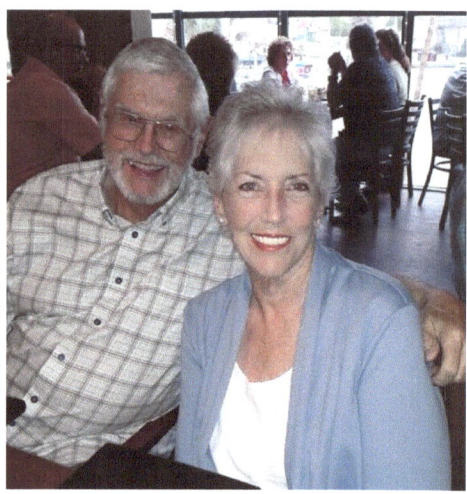

So far, I'm one of the lucky ones. As I write this, it has been almost a year since my first knee replacement was removed, but I am now able to walk with my new appliance … (sort of a hobble wobble) and my blood tests are stellar, because I am only eating things that are good for me. I drink high protein drinks, do not eat anything with processed sugar, (cakes, cookies, ice cream, etc.) take a multitude of vitamins and feel as though in writing this I am paying it forward.

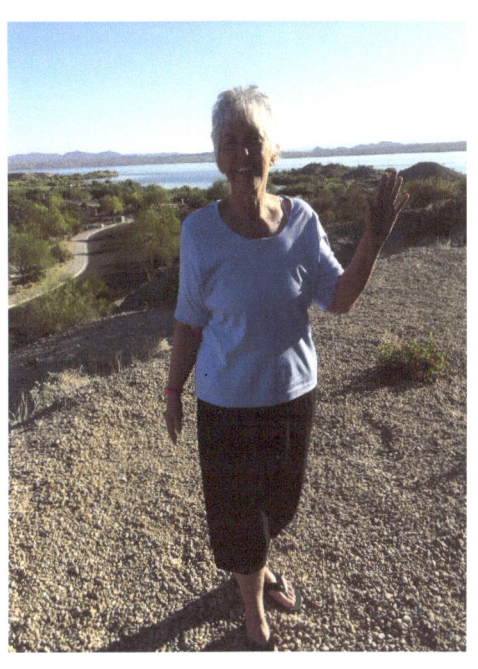

I hope this helps guide you in your decision. I don't want to scare you, and I would rather not be writing this, because it has brought back memories of the entire nightmare.

But if it helps you get the nerve up to have a frank conversation with your surgeon about the risks, and what that person can do to help you guard against going through anything like this, then it's been worth it.

So, if, after reading all of this extremely scary information, you decide to go ahead with your replacement here are the things you can expect with your brand new knee: (Not all of these things will necessarily apply to you, but a lot of them are possible)

Expect to loose sleep after you get home from the hospital due to:

- Pain in your cut muscles

- Not being able to roll over

- Not being able to lift your leg without using a strap

- Pain from physical therapy sessions

- Electrical shocks when the nerves in your muscles reattach. It hurts, but it means you are healing.

- Pain meds work, but may constipate you.

- Take fiber every day.

- Try to wean yourself off of the meds as soon as you can, yet when using them try to stay ahead of the pain.

- Remember that everything you put in your body goes through your liver. Drink lots of water, even though it requires more trips and hurts to walk to the bathroom.

Things to Buy, Rent, Do's & Don'ts

- Do <u>not</u> shave for a minimum of a week before your surgery.

- Wash your leg with a prescription anti-bacterial soap for several days before the surgery.

- Have a grab bar installed near your toilet and in your shower.

- Before surgery, place chairs strategically throughout your home, so you can rest.

- Rent or buy a raised commode that can fit over your toilet.

- Use a step to get into bed

- Use a shower seat and put down a non-slip shower mat inside your shower.

- Use a walker at first, then maybe a cane, depending on your balance capability.

- If you don't live with someone who can help you, hire a caregiver.

- Keep track of your meds. When you are drugged for pain, you can easily loose track and take too much.

- Only you know how much pain you are in.

- Take care of your incision. Watch it carefully for infection. Tape a Kotex or something like it over it to protect it from rubbing your sheets or pants.

- Wear loose fitting pants and be sure to rinse them at least one extra time when you wash them to get rid of soap residue.

- Use frozen and cold gel packs. Put them under your knee. That's where the blood flows the most.

- The very best exercise you can do is a sit to stand. Do as many as you can.

- Exercise bikes...

  A recumbent is the kind you sit on with your feet out on front, or a regular stationary bike allows you to sit up with your feet in a downward position. Your physical therapist can help you decide. But whatever you decide, be sure to use it. It will help your muscles remember to stretch back out.

- Walk heel to toe. Stand up straight. Try not to limp.

- Think about every step.

- If you drop something, let it fall. Re-read this sentence.

- Wear a Fitbit or use an iPhone to track your distances each day. It will help you encourage yourself to go farther.

- Make yourself get up to answer the phone. Even if all you do is stand.

- Keep your feet up, but lift your leg up from wherever you have it propped in revolutions of six every half hour.

- Never let your knee act as a bridge. Always try to support it with an ottoman or your mattress or on your sofa.

- Watch or read something interesting, so you forget about yourself.

- In the first week or two you will want to lie in bed... But try to prop yourself up as much as possible.

- Practice breathing exercises: Take a deep breath, hold it to a count of twelve, then breathe it out hard. Do that three times... This will loosen phlegm...

- Use that plastic breathing thing (that's the technical term) that they send you home with from the hospital. It would be horrible to go through the surgery and then die of pneumonia, just because you were stubborn or didn't think you needed to use it.

- When you want to turn around, take several small steps... Don't try to spin.

- Don't get cocky trying to keep up with family and friends if you go somewhere... Go as slow as you need to... They will wait and even escort you. I have found that 98% of the general population are kind and try to be careful around limping people... but there's always going to be that 2% that are in their own world, in a hurry and simply don't see you. Those are the ones you have to watch out for, because you can get knocked flat in an instant.

- Whatever it is you decide to do, about your surgery, be sure to keep your immune system up!!!! Do not eat sugar... It feeds bacteria.

- A couple of last things: if you throw up on your physical therapist they'll forgive you. They keep changes of clothes at the hospital, because people throw up on them every day.

- And lastly, laugh every day.
At one point, when I was in the long-term care facility, I had scooted over onto the commode and a man walked into the room. He sat in one of the guest chairs holding some papers and began to talk to me regarding whatever was on them.

I held up my hand and asked him if we could get together a little later on and he figured out where I was sitting, said "oh, I'm sorry, I'll be back later, when do you think you'll be done?" I cried I laughed so hard. I still have no clue who he was, what he wanted to talk about, and I never saw him again.

So, try to throw stress out of the window and see the humor in everyday life.

Here's my email address, just in case you want to ask me any non-medical questions:

Boyer.barbara@icloud.com

Thank you so much for buying the book.

Barb

Laugh

Relax

Breathe

And have a real conversation
with your Doctor (s).

www.ingramcontent.com/pod-product-compliance
Lightning Source LLC
Chambersburg PA
CBHW050928290526
45792CB00002B/928